A Parents 5 Step Guide to Lead Poisoning

From the Series

Lead Paint Clear and Simple

Book 1

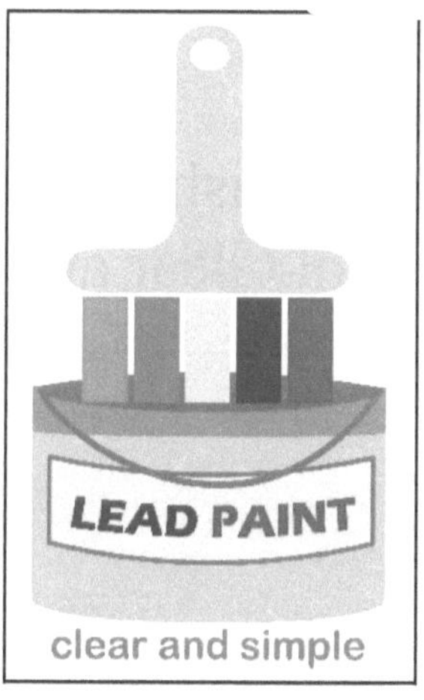

Kate Kirkwood

Copyright

Published by
Lead Paint Clear and Simple

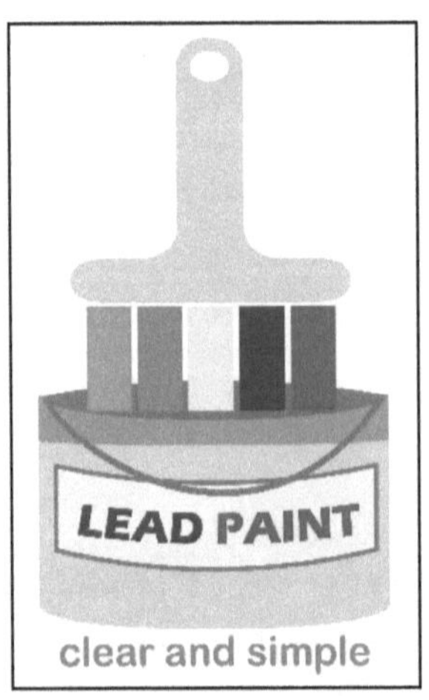

Forward

Many years ago, as a college business professor, a mentor of mine asked me "Do you want to teach? Or do you want to help people learn? They are not the same." I have been learning, teaching, training and working in the world of lead paint hazards, cleanup and regulations for about 15 years now, and I think it continues to get more cumbersome and more confusing every day. No one's fault really. It is an evolving problem, science and industry, with too many players, opinions, and egos. The federal government does their part, the States do their part, private industry contributes trainers, contractors and landlords, local code enforcement chimes in, the medical profession, and parents try to do what is best for the children.

Having worked as a grant writer, program/project manager, trainer, lead abatement contractor, risk assessor, lead inspector, intake specialist, certified renovator, healthy homes rater, dust sampling technician, outreach coordinator and consultant – I think I have seen it from most (perhaps not all) angles, and I humbly offer these suggestions to parents and caregivers who seek to understand how to keep kids safe. Following books in the series will attempt to offer simple and positive solutions to contractors, landlords, and other participants in this industry. In the end – do no harm. Test the people (blood) and the houses and strive to keep both clear of the invisible poisonous dust. I hope this little book will help make it more clear and simple, which will make it easier to learn.

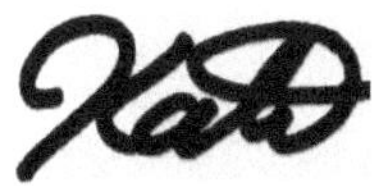

Table of Contents

Introduction

The truth about lead poisoning

Perhaps you bought this book because you live in an old home, built before 1978, or 1778 - or you care about a child who lives in an old home, or attends daycare, preschool or some other activities in old buildings. You have heard about lead poisoning and you are worried about the child.

It's a good thing to worry about. Evidence indicates that 1.2 million American children are now or have been lead poisoned, and we are only treating ½ of them.[1]

What does that mean, exactly? Do they have permanent disabilities? Maybe. Lead is a factor in many childhood concerns like ADHD, learning disabilities and confusion with and diagnosis of autism.[2]

Get Your Free Gift.......See Page 54

For more information check out our list of websites and resources at the end of this book.

I know you want to know whether the child in your life might be lead poisoned, but first, I want to direct your attention to your own activities. Are you lead poisoned? How about other adults in the child's life?

I wonder about that not only for you and your own health, but also to point out to you that adults who live or work around lead paint or dust, might also bring this dust home to their children or grandchildren, and this could even be the cause of the youngster's high lead levels.

So, much like the airlines, who tell you that in case of an emergency you should take care of your own oxygen mask before tending to the child sitting next to you – let's start by looking at your relationship to lead paint and lead poisoning.

Part One

Am I Lead Poisoned?

Have you ever scraped and painted an old house? Even just a room or two? Refurbished old furniture you bought at an antique shop or a yard sale? Worked in an auto repair shop? Refinished a boat? Spent time on a firing range or working on stained glass, painted china or canvas?

You might be lead poisoned yourself!

Imagine that while you are working with this material you don't realize that tiny little bits of dust and debris or paint chips are scraped or rubbed from your project and are on your clothes, or under your fingernails, and they fall to the floor and are ground into dust under your feet. Maybe you don't know that this is a highly toxic substance and that in fact an amount smaller than a granule of sugar is enough to poison you and to affect the way your brain works.

Get Your Free Gift.......See Page 54

If you were to "forget" to use your respirator, or set up your air cleaning system, perhaps you might breathe in some of these substances while you're working.

If I came to visit you while you were working, and I tossed a box of donuts on the table perhaps you'd eat one without stopping to wash your hands? If so, is it possible that a little bit of lead dust which might be on your hands, or under your fingernails, might get transferred to that donut, and find its way into your stomach? Or maybe I might come in and bring you a sandwich for lunch and you might be hungry, and there might not be water readily available to wash so you just sit down and eat. Maybe you would wipe your hands on your jeans, which are also covered with the same lead chips and dust.

Yes, lead poisoning happens to adults as well.

What are some of the symptoms of adult lead poisoning? Headaches, high blood pressure, memory loss, sexual dysfunction, joint pain, digestive problems, and increasing rates of miscarriage.[3]

Get Your Free Gift.......See Page 54

In fact, many adults that we have worked with, once they discovered that they had an elevated lead level and did some things to bring their lead level back down, felt better than they have felt in decades. Not knowing about adult lead poisoning, they thought they were seeing symptoms of diabetes, arthritis, obesity, or just general aging. They were amazed to find that reducing the lead level reduced the symptoms as well.

Does any of this sound familiar? Do you think that you could be lead poisoned? It's easy to find out! You can go to any Doctor's office, or any lab or any hospital or any health department and request a "quick test" for lead. There is a machine available in many of these locations called the "lead care II" [4] which allows a technician to give you a capillary test. It is a quick test, which is a finger prick, much like a diabetic checking for sugar. You can learn your blood lead level in 3 minutes from this test, and insurance will cover it (so will Medicaid and Medicare), so why not find out? By the way, your kids can have the same quick test – but more about that later.

This test will not check for "old" lead poisoning. Our blood refreshes every few weeks, so we are only testing for lead exposure in the last couple of months. The most likely adults who are lead poisoned are people who work or live in a building built before 1978. The older the building, the more likely there will be lead. The department of Housing and Urban Development (HUD) says that 9 out of 10 houses built before 1940 contain lead paint.[5]

HU Characteristic	All HUs (000)	Number of HUs[a] with LBP (000)			Percent of HUs[b] with LBP (%)			HUs in Sample
		Estimate	Lower 95% CI[c]	Upper 95% CI	Estimate	Lower 95% CI	Upper 95% CI	
Total Housing Units[a]	95,688	37,897	34,521	41,272	40%	36%	43%	831
	106,033	37,058	34,047	40,068	34.9%	32.1%	37.8%	1,131
Region:								
Northeast	19,290	10,600	8,306	12,895	55%	46%	64%	155
	20,190	10,121	8,722	11,519	50.1%	43.3%	57.0%	196
Midwest	22,083	11,748	10,546	12,950	53%	48%	59%	196
	23,994	9,358	7,924	10,791	39.0%	33.4%	44.6%	245
South	35,474	9,607	7,762	11,451	27%	22%	32%	277
	38,996	11,003	9,114	12,892	28.2%	23.2%	33.3%	440
West	18,841	5,942	4,747	7,137	32%	25%	38%	203
	22,853	6,576	5,345	7,808	28.8%	23.8%	33.8%	250
Construction Year:								
1978-1998	29,775	2,031	687	3,373	7%	2%	11%	220
1978-2005	40,458	2,675	1,458	3,893	6.6%	3.6%	9.6%	476
1960-1977	27,874	6,577	4,875	8,280	24%	18%	30%	267
	29,956	7,376	5,761	8,991	24.6%	19.5%	29.8%	306
1940-1959	20,564	14,171	12,203	16,139	69%	60%	77%	186
	18,117	11,921	10,645	13,197	65.8%	58.6%	73.0%	187
Before 1940	17,476	15,117	13,532	16,702	87%	82%	91%	158
	17,502	15,085	13,932	16,239	86.2%	79.7%	92.7%	162

Table ES-1. Prevalence of Lead-Based Paint (LBP) in AHHS (red) by Region and Housing Unit (HU) Age, with Comparisons to NSLAH (Statistically Significant Differences Highlighted)

[a] "Housing units" include permanently occupied, noninstitutional housing units in which children are permitted to live.
[b] All percentages are calculated with the "all HUs" on the left most column of each row as the denominator.
[c] CI = confidence interval for the estimated number or percent.

Get Your Free Gift.......See Page 54

Some people think that lead is a problem that we took care of many years ago. We banned lead in gasoline in the 70's right? Didn't that solve the problem? Well, it did take care of a big part of the "lead burden" in our country, but there are more issues.

People think we outlawed lead in house paint, but that's not really true. The federal government outlawed the manufacture of lead-based paint for residential use in 1978. However, you could still buy the paint, and you could still use it if you had it, so houses built for several years after 1978 can have lead in them. Also, even if you painted over the lead with latex paint many times the fact is that lead paint is still underneath it. So as the latex paint chips away or we scrape it to repaint, or drill a hole in it to install cable, or hang a painting, the lead reappears, and little bits of that lead get into your blood and into your stomach, and lungs, and brain.

There are only two ways that we get lead poisoned as far as we know today. We must eat or breathe in the chips or dust. If we breathe it in, then it's in our lungs and passes through the lining of our lungs into our bloodstream. In fact, if we breathe in vapors (from the melting or burning of the lead) those fumes can go directly to our brain and poison us much more quickly. That was the big problem with leaded gasoline – which, by the way, is still in use today in some heavy equipment and farm vehicles.

When we eat the lead (from our hands or what has got into our food or drinks while we work around lead dust) it gets into our stomach and passes through the lining of our stomach as it is digested and then into our bloodstream, where it's carried to our brain.

I want to point out that the smaller the particle of lead, the more dangerous it is. Without getting too graphic, you could eat a paint chip, or a chunk of lead and it could pass through you and pretty much come out in the shape in which it went in right? (ewwwww, gross……) But, an amount of dust too small to see is breathed in or eaten and there is no way to keep from absorbing that into our blood stream and eventually it will work its way to our brain.

Another way that adults get lead poisoned has to do with our hobbies and activities. For example, let's say you paint on canvas or china or any other substance. You might do beautiful work and give these items as gifts or sell them at craft fairs.

If you buy an artist quality paint, maybe at the mall, or on line, read the label of that tube of paint. It very likely contains lead. Artist paint is not regulated with regard to lead content.

Get Your Free Gift.......See Page 54

Maybe you repair your own cars or boats. Because one of the qualities of lead paint is that it inhibits rust, mold and mildew, it is frequently used in automotive paints and is a very important ingredient in marine paints. Do you spend any time at an indoor firing range? Maybe you have heard that California has banned the use of lead bullets? [6] In fact, in 1989, Thomas Kelly, a 35-year-old police sergeant in the Derry, NH police force, died because of the lead level in his blood from spending so much time in indoor firing ranges.[7]

Do you own or renovate older homes? Some people, who know about the dangers of lead paint, believe that clear varnish and stain are not affected. In fact, the newest EPA regulation, the Renovate, Repair and Paint Rule (RRP) [8] clearly identifies "paint and surface coatings" as the issue because stain might have lead in it too, and there were additives to some varnish to help it dry quickly. So, you have to check the varnished woodwork just like the painted woodwork – and later in this book, I will give you the options for how to check.

Many dishes and household items, including toys, contain lead.[9]

One of the problems is that some countries do not have the same regulations that we have in the United States, (where I am based), with regard to lead and therefore it is not unusual to find lead in toys and furniture.

Visit our Facebook page https://www.facebook.com/leadedu or website at http://www.lead-edu.info and you'll see recalls on such things as baby cribs, baby food, formula and toys.

When you are repairing or updating something old, do you wear any kind of personal protection? At the very least, pick up a disposable respirator that is rated for lead. That would be the 100 series. N100, R100, P100; or get a reusable ½ face with changeable cartridges (purple, or magenta, is the color for lead) and when you buy one, ask about having it "fit tested" to be sure it is working correctly.

When you are renovating an older home or anywhere you believe that you may have come in contact with lead dust then you need to wash carefully, not just your hands and your clothing, but everything that you touched or anyplace that's dusty from your work.

Get Your Free Gift.......See Page 54

Also, if you are doing the work in the US for "compensation" – someone is paying you or you are increasing or maintaining the value of an investment, then you need to know about the EPA's RRP rule.

This rule is called "renovate repair and paint" (RRP) and it took effect in April of 2010. The bottom line is it says you must take an 8-hour lead paint safety certification class if you are doing any activities that disturb Lead-Based paint in a home or commercial child occupied facility. These classes are available in the US for around $200 per person and will certify you for 5 years.

When you get this training, you will learn that you must use containment, which means use duct tape to hold plastic in place so that the chips and dust are collected there and can be thrown away. If you are making a lead mess by sanding and scraping old paint, make it in as small an area as possible and then you must use very detailed cleaning methods when you finish the job to be sure no bits of dust remain.

Get Your Free Gift.......See Page 54

Broom-clean is a thing of the past! What we are doing now is washing everything that may have been contaminated by this dust, and we are using a special vacuum with a filter that is the correct size to catch the lead. It's called a HEPA vacuum, and it has a filter that is 99.97% effective at .3 microns. The vacuum is not just one with the correct filter, but it also must be a "sealed unit" meaning that there are gaskets everyplace that the vacuum opens or comes apart. That way no dust can get out because the air must pass through the filter before it is exhausted to the outside. A shop vac with a HEPA filter is NOT sufficient!

Lastly, we are throwing away the rags that we used to wash the surfaces so that we do not re-contaminate them by spreading the lead dust around the way we would if we used a mop or a sponge. Disposable rags should be purchased, or you can make your own with paper towels and any soap.

One of my companies provides the RRP training class, and I often teach it myself, so I can tell you we spend a lot of time talking about how to contain the dust. We spend 8 hours talking about lead safety and cleaning in a much more detailed way. There is a video that will help to understand this, and you can access it by going to www.youtube.com and search "EPA contractor Kevin Sheehan" or click here

https://www.youtube.com/watch?v=4UTRE0QeUs4

Get Your Free Gift.......See Page 54

This video features my friend, Kevin Sheehan who said "it's like the difference between washing your car and detailing your car"….it's a different kind of clean.

There are some simple solutions that you can implement when you strive to keep your world lead-safe. For example, if you work in a place where you think you might carry lead dust home, just take your shoes off before you walk into your house at the end of your work day.

Another example is to think about the lead dust that might be in your car, and perhaps keep a separate vehicle for the family to use and make your "work vehicle" just that – keeping the dust away from the kids.

There was a study done in 2008 in the state of Maine called the infant car seat study.[10] There were some children in ME, who were lead poisoned and there was no easy answer as to why. In other words, they were not living in older homes, or spending their days in older buildings, yet these kids had elevated blood lead levels.

Get Your Free Gift…….See Page 54

An investigation pointed out the fact that there were high levels of leaded dust in the entryways to their buildings, even though the buildings were new, so it was obviously brought in from somewhere.

That led investigators to try looking outside the house and they found high lead levels on the front porches or the steps and in the driveways. So that led them to check the vehicles that were parked in the driveway.

It turned out in this investigation that parents were responsible for bringing lead dust into the house and their vehicles had very high lead concentrations. The saddest part of the story is that the highest lead levels were in the infant car seats in the back of the pickup trucks.

We can understand how this happens, right? Mom or dad drops the baby off at day care on the way to work in the morning, and for the rest of the day, if you are working in painting or construction or renovation - what happens in that back seat? Coats, tools, drop-cloths.....all sorts of things that are covered with dust (and now we know poisonous dust) are in the back of this vehicle. At the end of the day, we push these things out of the way, and pop junior into his car seat, where he is exposed to this lead dust all the way home from work.

Get Your Free Gift.......See Page 54

Very sad, very common, and completely avoidable.

Once you understand what you are dealing with, you will come up with a solution that will work for you.

Perhaps it will be a different vehicle for your family's use as opposed to the work vehicle. Perhaps it will mean someone else driving to daycare. Perhaps it will be a separate "work" bathroom where you come in the house and wash and change clothes to get rid of the lead before you hug the kids.

Parents, even if you live in a new home, you must be aware of "take home lead" This is the subject of a TEDX Wilmington talk planned for shortly after this book is published and scheduled to be presented in May of 2018. Perhaps by the time you are reading this book, you can search for the talk on youtube – given by the author and learn more about the lead hazards that can exist in NEW homes.

Get Your Free Gift.......See Page 54

If you live in a new home, but you work around old paint and you, yourself are lead poisoned. Because you are an adult, we can bring your lead level back down to normal and the symptoms of lead poisoning will largely disappear. But what you bring home to your child has a very different effect on them. More info on that in Part 2 of this book.

The other potential danger for children is the house in which they live. Maybe, you don't need to bring lead home with you, maybe it's already in the house. If you live in an older home with paint that is peeling, chipping and flaking, regardless of how many times you repaint the inside of your house with latex, the lead paint is still there. So, when you chip the paint with furniture moving or bumping into it with a sharp object, there is lead dust on the floor.

Also, if you are working inside a home and you cut, sand, drill, scrape or in some way disturb paint in that home you are creating little bits of poisonous dust added to the regular household dust on the floor.

Sometimes the dust is just from living in the home. For instance, you might have an old window which opens and closes with friction between the sash and the casing of the window. The wood becomes bare, as the paint is scraped off. Little bits of lead dust have rubbed off the window itself or the casing – Where is that paint now? That dust and paint was made up of lead – it didn't disappear – so what happened to it?

Well, lead is heavy – so, gravity does its job, lead falls down and it ends up in the window well and on the window sill. Some might fall on the floor, and when the window is opened those little bits blow all over the house, and they collect in the cracks in the floorboards, or in the corners.

Another source of lead dust is doors. When the door is first installed, it is square and flush with the casing, and it opens and closes without rubbing or catching anywhere. After a while, the house settles and wood swells and pretty soon the door sticks and you have to "hip check" it to close it and yank on it to open it.

Get Your Free Gift.......See Page 54

Now look at the edge of that door and you will see the paint is worn off and there is bare wood showing. Once again – where did those bits of lead go? They are not "gone". In the carpet? On the floor? Then they were tracked where?

Since lead dust is heavy, it's not like asbestos that stays suspended in the air for a long time. In fact, if we stirred up a bunch of lead dust in the room you are sitting in now, within about an hour, all that dust would settle out of the air, and gravity would cause it to settle down onto the floor, or the counter, or any horizontal surface.

To further complicate this situation, when the child is a baby we are told by the Doctor and other child care experts that the safest place to put the baby is on the floor. In fact, they encourage us to put the baby down for "blanket time" or "floor time" or "tummy time" or whatever your professional calls it. It makes sense, right? They can't fall off the floor like they can from a bed or couch, and they can stretch and ultimately roll over and learn to use their muscles. So, we put them on the floor. Given the option of 2 floors – you will choose the one with carpet over a bare floor.

However, now we know they are lying in a collection of toxic dust from the lead, and if you chose carpet – that's even worse, as the lead dust gets trapped in the carpet fibers. If you look around the room you are sitting in now, you will see what I mean. There are little bits of dust and debris everywhere! Under the furniture and on the window sill for example.

I don't mean your house is dirty. The dust we are talking about can be too small to see. It can be like the little particles in the air we see when the sunlight streams through the window, or that raises when we hit the couch cushions.

When that child starts to crawl around, their hands will be on the floor and in the dust all the time. The dust will be on their toys, their sippy cups, pacifiers, bottles, and snacks. They will have ample opportunity to eat the dust, as well as breathe it in, which, of course, is the problem. This is called "hand-to-mouth behavior" and all babies and toddlers do this.

Another factor is that stuffed animals can be covered in these little bits of dust and then that animal gets snuggled, kissed, hugged and played with all day long and sleeps with the child at night giving the child extra opportunities to breathe in the dust.

Get Your Free Gift.......See Page 54

Sometimes pets roll in the dirt in the yard, or the lead dust on the windows and then come over to snuggle or play with your toddler and they could be exposing them to lead dust at the same time.

You don't know by looking at it if that dust has lead in it, but if the house is built between 1960 and 1978, 1 out of 4 houses will contain lead – and if it's built before 1940 then 9 out of 10 will have lead in the dust.[5]

If the outside of the house was painted with lead, that paint might be chipping and peeling on the porch, and you might be tracking it into the house. Sometimes the chips fall off the house and contaminate the soil around the drip line. That soil might get tracked into the house too.

What if you just don't know? Is there lead in your house or not? How can you tell?

There are a couple of ways to find out. If you contact your department of health and human services and/or childhood lead poisoning prevention program generally located in the State capital at the State offices, they will be able to help you. See how to reach them by going to this note (number 11) at the end of the book [11]

When you contact the program in your State, ask them for a list of certified lead inspectors. Lead Inspectors will come to your home with an XRF instrument where they can "shoot" any painted surface, and without damaging the surface get a "reading" of how much lead is there. They will be able to read through several layers of latex paint, or through sheetrock, or paneling and identify where the lead is "underneath" a covering.

Why would you care? I mean, if it's under the latex we are safe, aren't we? Well, what if you hit the latex paint with a toy or a tool or a piece of furniture and expose the lead underneath it? What if the sheetrock is damaged by a water leak and deteriorates? Lots of things can "re-expose" you, and your children to the lead underneath including, of course, renovation.

Get Your Free Gift.......See Page 54

If you want more help – ask for a list of Risk Assessors. These folks are more experienced and trained and have additional certification beyond that of a lead inspector. So, they can not only test the surfaces, but they can also, as you might imagine "assess the risk".

A Risk Assessor will tell you what they think should be done with each of the leaded surfaces, within your State's (and EPA's) regulations that will make the property lead safe. If you, or a contractor, completes that work in a safe way, the same risk assessor can come back and inspect to let you know that the property is safe now, and you can get a certificate that says so.

However, if you just want a quick idea about whether there is lead in your home, you can also contact a "dust sampling technician" (DST). All they can do is collect dust wipes and send the wipes to a lab to be analyzed. Sometimes, that's enough!

If there is a lead hazard in your home, there will be lead in the dust on your floor and window sills. So, if you hire a DST and have them take a few samples, you will have a good idea whether you have a problem with lead hazards in your house. These professionals do not have expensive equipment, such as an XRF, and less training is required for their certification, so they are less expensive to hire.

When you are having a renovation done be sure to hire an RRP (renovate repair and paint) EPA/HUD certified contractor.[12] If you are using the EPA locator to find a renovator please note that there are 15 locations (shown at the top of the locator page) that manage this rule themselves, and therefore you must click on those links to find someone in that state. However, if you scroll down further, you will see the national search database for everywhere else. Once you find a lead safe renovator, they will test the components they are working on by using a recognized test kit like "lead check" or "d-lead" so you will know if there is lead in any of the paint they are disturbing.

Get Your Free Gift.......See Page 54

You CANNOT ask them to test the whole house, though, unless they are also certified as lead inspectors, or risk assessors. The RRP rule only allows them to test those components that they are renovating. A lead inspector has a lot more training to be sure they don't miss anything, and will test the whole house (inside, outside, dust and soil). Renovators are just going to test the parts of the house they are working on.

As a homeowner, or landlord, you can take the RRP class too, and you will learn a lot about the dangers of lead and how to handle it safely. In fact, landlords are required to take the class if they do their own work (disturbing paint) at tenant change over. If you are a landlord and don't do your own work, but hire someone, be sure they are RRP or State certified.

If you just bought one of the lead testing kits at the hardware store and have not taken any classes, but you want to use them yourself, you should know that most people do not use them correctly. There are some instructional videos on the web at different sites, including **http://www.lead-edu.info/helpful-videos** so be sure, before you use them that you understand the way they work and their limitations. They are a great tool, and even as a Lead Inspector/Risk Assessor myself, I still used them in some situations, and I teach other people to use them.

Get Your Free Gift.......See Page 54

I have even seen people make up a sort of Do-it-yourself "dust wipe" by taking a wet paper towel and picking up some dust on the floor, then dripping the liquid from a lead check swab onto the dust to see if it turns red. Now this is not recognized anywhere as a dust wipe, but it will let you know if there is lead in the dust. Once you know that there is lead dust, you might decide to take a course, or hire a professional to get more information.

At the end of this book there are a number of web sites and links that can help you find the right person in your state who might be able to help you get more information, and you can also feel free to contact my office. Although we are located in New Hampshire, we have access to information about every State and their resources.[11]

Now, let's move to the second part of this book and talk about the kids.

Part Two

Is My Child Lead Poisoned?
How would I know?

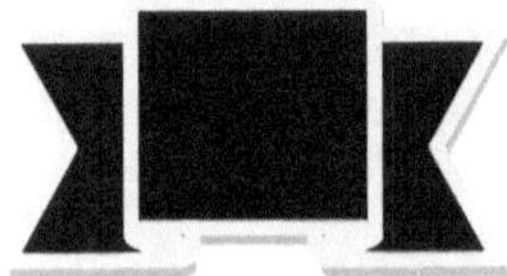

Get your child tested! There is only one way to know if your child is lead poisoned and that is to have a blood test done. The simplest test is a capillary "finger stick" test. This was discussed in section one of this book and is like a diabetic checking for sugar.

The equipment used to provide this test is called the Lead Care II machine [4] and it is readily available. Results will be provided within 3 minutes, and although it is not as accurate as a more standard blood test, it is a great screening tool.

If your level, or your child's level comes back elevated, it will be recommended that you should have a venous draw, which is a more traditional blood test.

Get Your Free Gift.......See Page 54

This standard test can be taken in conjunction with other blood work, and results will be available within a few days.

Lead in the blood is measured in micrograms per deciliter (µg/dl) and the Center for Disease Control's (CDC's) current level of concern, as of 2018, is 5 µg/dl.

Many states have a level of action of 10 µg/dl, but this is too high! If your child has a level of 10 µg/dl, damage is already occurring. Do not accept the technician or the Doctor's office just giving you unilateral assurance that the child is fine, or that the level is normal, ask for a number. You want to make sure that that number is less than five.

Also, be aware that the quick test machine cannot measure below 3.3 µg/dl, so when a child's level shows up as "low" on the lead care II machine that simply means that the level is lower than 3.3 µg/dl.

When your child's blood test is done by venous draw, the results are more specific and accurate.

Get Your Free Gift.......See Page 54

What happens when a child is lead poisoned?

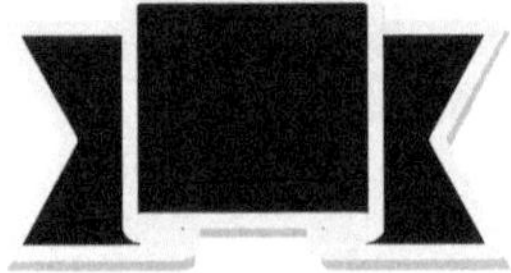

The sad thing about childhood lead poisoning is it interferes with the neurological pathways in their brain. Children, up to age six, are in the developmental stage and their brain is functioning on a fast track for learning.

When you go to the doctor's office with a child who is 12 months old, they give you a developmental chart for a 12-month-old. When you go with a child who is 18 months old, they will give you a different developmental chart. This chart lets you check off which things your child is doing and compare your child's development to the standard for that age.

We can do this because we know when the developmental milestones should have occurred in a child's brain and when they should be able to complete certain functions and processes.

Get Your Free Gift.......See Page 54

Because of this kind of research, we can identify that some lead poisoned children have lower IQ's then non-poisoned kids, some have permanent brain damage, and some will develop behavioural problems like ADHD, hearing loss, speech disorders and other symptoms.[13]

Further research indicates that children who are lead poisoned have a greater likelihood of ending up in a special education program, earning less money than average, are more likely to spend time in juvenile detention facilities, and later in prison as a violent criminal.[14]

No child has to be lead poisoned! It is, in fact, one of the most preventable childhood diseases, and that makes it doubly tragic.

Hear it from Ralph Spezio, whose TedX talk is available on YouTube. You can access it by going to www.youtube.com and searching "Ralph Spezio TedX talk" or just click here https://www.youtube.com/watch?v=mSwHSE6_Zo I

Dr Sprzio's talk tells the story of a small elementary school in Rochester New York where the children's test scores were not acceptable, and their work was below required standards.

After looking into several other possible reasons, the school tested the children for elevated lead in their blood.

It was determined that 42% of the children in this small neighborhood school had an elevated blood lead level, but that's not even the tragic statistic. Dr. Spezio's team identified the fact that in his special education programs, 100% of the children had an elevated blood lead level!

Most states are not testing the majority of the children. It is not standard at the pediatrician's office when you take your children for immunizations and well-baby visits. Even though the American Academy of Pediatrics has recommended that all children should be tested at age one and age two, this is seldom a part of the routine practice of pediatricians.[15]

So, if you take nothing else from this little book, please get every child under six in your life tested! It's quick, it's easy, and it's not expensive

One of the reasons that we have so many lead poisoned children, is that the symptoms of lead poisoning are not easily identifiable. The child is poisoned by breathing or eating the little tiny bits of dust in their house, daycare, or other building where they spend a significant amount of time. When the child first encounters this toxin, do you know what happens?

They cough or sneeze, and they have a runny nose. That's what your body does to get rid of dust and substances that it does not like that you have breathed in, It makes mucus and causes you to cough or sneeze to get rid of the dust.

Who even notices a toddler with a runny nose? That's just a part of their life isn't it?

And what about the child who is further poisoned and begins to show signs of violent behavior? If you see a two-year-old throw a toy, hit a child, or scream out in anger… What do you think is happening? Terrible twos? They really need a timeout? Perhaps. Or perhaps we are beginning to see the violent behavior that so often accompanies lead poisoning.[16]

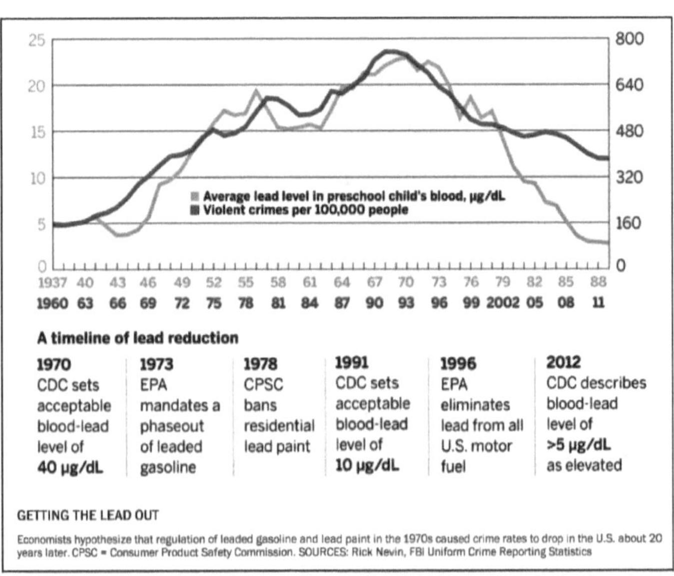

A timeline of lead reduction

1970	**1973**	**1978**	**1991**	**1996**	**2012**
CDC sets acceptable blood-lead level of **40 µg/dL**	EPA mandates a phaseout of leaded gasoline	CPSC bans residential lead paint	CDC sets acceptable blood-lead level of **10 µg/dL**	EPA eliminates lead from all U.S. motor fuel	CDC describes blood-lead level of **>5 µg/dL** as elevated

GETTING THE LEAD OUT

Economists hypothesize that regulation of leaded gasoline and lead paint in the 1970s caused crime rates to drop in the U.S. about 20 years later. CPSC = Consumer Product Safety Commission. SOURCES: Rick Nevin, FBI Uniform Crime Reporting Statistics

Get Your Free Gift…….See Page 54

What do I do if they do have high lead levels?

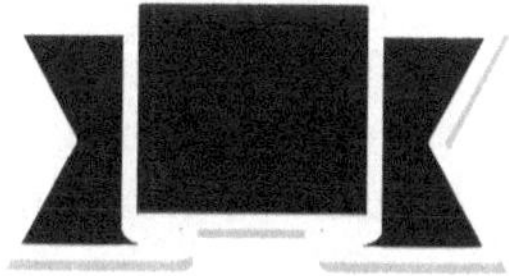

Work with your doctor to schedule regular blood lead level tests and be sure the level is going down.

Clean up any lead dust in the house with a HEPA vacuum and wet disposable cloths.

Make sure the home is lead safe (no chipping peeling paint). Just cover it. Paint all deteriorated surfaces. Even if you just paint them over with latex paint – that's better than leaving the chips and dust accessible to the children. Now, I'm not suggesting that painting them over with latex is a long-term solution. It is not! However, it's a great band aid – particularly if you plan to abate later.

It is important to stop here and explain that there is a HUGE difference between renovation and lead abatement.

Renovation means remodeling, improving, or making a property better in some way. It could be anything from touching up paint, to replacing a window, to gutting the whole house. The point is to make it worth more, or look better, or be more modern, or more comfortable. The reason is to update, or perhaps to sell or rent.

Any lead paint that is disturbed during renovation is incidental – the renovator tests and knows it is there, works carefully when dealing with it – but it's not the focus of the work. Hire RRP certified contractors or get certified if you will do the work yourself. This is called "lead safe renovation" and this law requires that you take the one day class and pass the test before doing work for "compensation" in a pre-78 building.

Abatement, on the other hand, means the permanent and complete removal or covering of all lead hazards on the property.   This would include all painted surfaces on the inside and outside of the property, AND all leaded dust and soil that may be identified as part of the process.

A lead abatement job, must be completed by a lead abatement certified contractor (as opposed to RRP), and the job starts with a lead inspection to identify where all the lead is located. EPA and/or State rules of abatement must be followed, and then at the end of the job a lead inspector comes in to check and "clear" the property. Abatement contractors have taken a three or four-day class, and are certified by the State or by the EPA as "Lead Abatement Contractors"

The intent of an abatement project is to make the property safe by permanently addressing the lead hazards. It is not necessary that the property look better or be improved when the abatement is done – but it is certainly safer.

Now, let's get back to what you can do to address lead levels. You can work to be sure the child or adult has a diet that will discourage the body from lead absorption. This should be a diet high in calcium, vitamin C and iron.[17] You should always wash hands before eating. Learn how to help your child by working with the contractor, school, parents, and doctors to form an effective team and keep them safe.[18]

How can we protect them, and ourselves?

Five steps, clear and simple

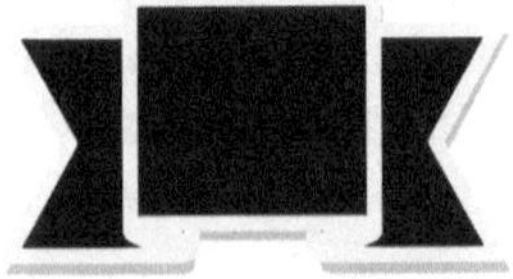

1) Test the kids

As mentioned earlier there are two ways to test kids (or adults) for an elevated blood lead level. You can have a quick test done, and you will have an approximate level between 3.3 µg/dl and 65 µg/dl.

Or you can have a venous draw, which is a more traditional blood test. In this case you'll have an accurate representation of the amount of lead in your blood at any level.

Get Your Free Gift.......See Page 54

Any amount of lead is dangerous! Certainly, take action if there is a lead level of 3.0 µg/dl or more. Go to your doctor, and read the information provided in the endnotes of this book. Visit our websites and Facebook pages – also listed at the end of this book, for additional information and tips.

2) Test the house

As we've discovered, there are several different ways to test the house.

The most thorough and complete way to do it is to hire a risk assessor.

The risk assessor will provide you with the complete report including all the surfaces in your house that contain lead paint, which ones have high risk, what the risk is, and what you should do about each of the surfaces. You will also have a number (mg/cm^2) to identify how much lead is in each location.

In some cases, you might have just a lead inspection done, and that would list the surfaces in the house that have lead, and how much lead is on each component.

You could also have just dust sampling done, and that will identify for you if there is lead dust on the floor and the windows in the house and it will tell you how much dust is where.

You can have a renovation contractor test just those components as a part of their specific renovation, but that does not identify any hazards in the rest of the house, and it does not give you an amount/quantity of lead – it's a yes/no test only.

You can purchase a recognized lead testing kit and do the testing yourself. In this case you will have no idea how much lead there is on any surface you'll just know if there is lead or there is no lead. For more information on this take an RRP class or watch the authors TEDX Wilmington talk.

3) **Raise awareness**

First, people must understand that we still have a problem with lead paint. That even though, in theory, at least, we stopped using it in 1978, it is still out there and still making kids sick.

Get Your Free Gift........See Page 54

Once they understand there is a problem then they have to understand how severe a problem it is, so we have to raise awareness about symptoms. Most people don't realize that lead dust robs kids of their IQ, earning potential, and in reality, their future.

At every opportunity literature has to be provided, presentations have to be given at schools, landlord meetings, general population gatherings such as rotary clubs, county fairs and other grassroots organizations Share this book, and the videos and resources in it.

Do you work in a school? There is ample evidence to indicate that in many communities a large percentage of the special education program children either are now or have been lead poisoned. Providing continuing education units (ceu's) for school nurses, and special education counsellors, can assist in both the prevention of lead poisoning for some children, and the best practices in terms of working with the lead poisoned child to achieve their full potential after damage has been done.

Landlords should be made aware of the need to provide "protect your family" books available at http://lead-edu.info/helpful-brochures on the sale or rental of the property, and "renovate right" books available at http://lead-edu.info/helpful-brochures on the renovation of the property.

Contractors must be certified and give out the renovate right book to all clients with property built before 1978.

Some members of the medical community may not be aware of the dangers of lead either. Often the doctors and nurses who trained many years ago, were not taught much about this hazard, so it is helpful to speak to your own doctors, and to arrange continuing education units for nurses, doctors, physicians' assistants, and community health specialist. In any case, ask your doctor for a blood test for you and your children, even if they don't think you need it. If you are worried, get the test!

4) Use lead safe practices around your home

When you recognize that there's lead in your house, you need to use a HEPA Vac for cleaning and wash all hard surfaces with disposable rags that get thrown away. If you use mops and buckets, or reusable sponges, you'll simply spread the lead dust around. Whereas, if you use disposable cloths, you will throw the lead away with each cloth and have much more success in your cleaning efforts.

Your HEPA Vac must be a sealed unit and must have a filter which is 99.97% effective at 0.3 microns, you must be careful when you are changing the bag that you do not deposit lead dust onto the carpet or into the air.

The best way to change the bag is to put down a small piece of plastic or a trash bag and work on the plastic making sure that no lead dust is released into the room and wear a respirator while changing the bag.

If you're going to do any home renovations, you should first test to see whether or not there is lead in the paint. If you are testing with a lead check swab, be sure you understand how to use them.

When using a lead check swab you must prepare the surface by cutting through any layers of paint on the wood. When you have sliced through the layers of paint down to the substrate you can drip the liquid from the lead check swab into the divot or hole or slice that you have made and if the liquid encounters lead at any level it will turn red.

You must also remember to drip your lead check swab on to the confirmation card to confirm that it is working correctly. Again – read the directions or watch the instructional video before using the swabs.

If you're using the d-lead kit follow the manufactures instructions carefully and put the lead chips, dust, or debris into the little glass vial along with five drops of the second chemical. Let it sit for 10 minutes, and then check the color of the liquid in the bottle against the standard. Remember before you dispose of the vial to dump it into the bag of crystals that came with the kit.

Check the expiration dates on the Dlead. There is no expiration on the lead check swabs, and they are freeze-thaw stable.

Get Your Free Gift.......See Page 54

If you are going to be scraping or sanding paint, do not use any power tools, unless they are attached to a HEPA Vac with a shroud or dust collecting device. It is permissible to hand scrape or sand, without power tools, however it would be wise to spray the area with water so that you are scraping or sanding wet instead of dry.

In all cases put down plastic and duct tape it to the floor so you can collect the dust and the debris into the plastic, and fold it dirty side in, corner to corner, and wrap it with duct tape for disposal in the dumpster.

If you are working in your primary residence, you do not need RRP certification however, of course you should have it, to keep your own family safe.

If you are working in a rental property, or a summer home, or an investment property, or someone is paying you to do this work, you must have the 8-hour RRP certification, which must be renewed every five years, or face fines of up to $37,500 per violation. To find an RRP class in your area go to
https://cfpub.epa.gov/flpp/pub/index.cfm?do=main .trainingSearch
or google and search "EPA RRP classes".

5) Hire lead certified contractors

If you're not going to do the work yourself, but you want to hire someone who's going to disturb paint on the inside or the outside of your home, or any building that you own that was built before 1978, where children go on a regular basis, you must hire a lead certified contractor.

These contractors should show you proof that they are EPA/HUD or State certified. In addition to this, the individual renovator should be working for a certified firm. That means they should also show you proof that their company has been certified by EPA/HUD or the state.

If you are the manager of a daycare, or a preschool, or any commercial building in which children under six congregate on a regular basis, the same rules apply to you as well.

Get Your Free Gift.......See Page 54

More "lead paint clear and simple" books are being created for contractors and landlords, this one is primarily for parents.

The contractor that you hire should be laying down plastic before disturbing any paint, they should never use a torch or a heat gun above 1100°, and they should never be using power tools to remove the old paint, unless the tools have a hose attached which directs all dust and debris into the HEPA Vac.

The bottom line is - no one poisons a child on purpose! However, we don't know what we don't know. Therefore, we don't always know what questions to ask.

Once people are aware of the problem most of us will function in integrity and do the right thing! But we can't do it if we don't know what it is.

You now have awareness of a terrible silent epidemic in America which is robbing our children of their potential. Please help to do your part to raise awareness, test children at every opportunity, and work lead safe.

Get Your Free Gift.......See Page 54

Endnotes and Resources

Lead Paint Clear and Simple
(http://leadpaintclearandsimple.com)

K. Kirkwood Consulting, LLC
(https://kkirkwood.com)

North East Health & Housing
(http://nehh.org)

Lead-Edu
(http://lead-edu.info)

Skylar Learns About Lead Poisoning
(http://www.skylarlearnsaboutleadpoisoning.com)

Lead Safe Mama
(http://www.leadsafemama.com)

[1] Sarah Frostenson, "1.2 million children in the US have lead poisoning. We're only treating half of them," Apr. 27, 2017
(https://www.vox.com/science-and-health/2017/4/27/15424050/us-underreports-lead-poisoning-cases-map-community).

[2] Tamara Rubin, "A Dad's Perspective; Autism Vs. Lead Poisoning," May 24, 2015
(http://tamararubin.com/2015/05/autism).

[3] U.S. Environmental Protection Agency, "Lead at

Get Your Free Gift.......See Page 54

Superfund Sites: Human Health"
(https://www.epa.gov/superfund/lead-superfund-sites-human-health).

[4] LeadCare II, "Frequently Asked Questions"
(http://www.leadcare2.com/Product-Support/FAQs).

[5] U.S. Department of Housing and Urban Development (HUD), Office of Healthy Homes and Lead Hazard Control, "American Healthy Homes Survey," Lead and Arsenic Findings, (April 2011), page ES-7 (https://www.hud.gov/sites/documents/AHHS_REPORT.PDF).

[6] California Department of Fish and Wildlife, "Nonlead Ammunition in California" (https://www.wildlife.ca.gov/hunting/nonlead-ammunition)

[7] Christine Willsmen, "Lead endangers officers," Apr. 10, 2015 (http://projects.seattletimes.com/2014/loaded-with-lead/4).

[8] U.S. Environmental Protection Agency, "Renovation, Repair and Painting Program" (https://www.epa.gov/lead/renovation-repair-and-painting-program).

[9] U.S. Environmental Protection Agency, "Lead in Toys and Toy Jewelry" (https://www.epa.gov/lead/lead-toys-and-toy-jewelry).

[10] Centers for Disease Control and Prevention, "Childhood Lead Poisoning Associated with Lead Dust Contamination

of Family Vehicles and Child Safety Seats," Maine, 2008 (https://www.cdc.gov/mmwr/preview/mmwrhtml/mm583 2a2.htm).

[11] Centers for Disease Control and Prevention, "State Programs" (https://www.cdc.gov/nceh/lead/programs/default.htm).

[12] Centers for Disease Control and Prevention, "Locate Certified Renovation and Lead Dust Sampling Technician Firms" (https://cfpub.epa.gov/flpp/pub/index.cfm?do=main.firm Search).

[13] All Things Considered, "Childhood Exposure To Lead Can Blunt IQ For Decades, Study Suggests," March 20, 2017 (https://www.npr.org/sections/health-shots/2017/03/28/521644395/study-suggests-childhood-exposure-to-lead-can-blunt-iq-for-decades).

[14] D. Amari Jackson, "Lead Astray: New Evidence Links Children with Higher Lead Exposure to School Suspensions and Juvenile Detention," June 27, 2017 (http://atlantablackstar.com/2017/06/27/lead-astray-new-evidence-links-children-higher-lead-exposure-school-suspensions-juvenile-detention).

[15] Joshua Schneyer and M.B. Pell, "Millions of American children missing early lead tests, Reuters finds," June 9, 2016 (https://www.reuters.com/investigates/special-report/lead-poisoning-testing-gaps).

[16] Kevin Drum, "An Updated Lead-Crime Roundup for 2018," Feb. 1, 2018

Get Your Free Gift........See Page 54

(https://www.motherjones.com/kevin-drum/2018/02/an-updated-lead-crime-roundup-for-2018).

[17] Bethany Thayer, MS, RDN, FAND, "How to Fight Lead Exposure with Nutrition," March 22, 2018 (https://www.eatright.org/health/wellness/preventing-illness/how-to-fight-lead-exposure-with-nutrition).

[18] Kathy Bishop and Julia Whitehead, "9 Ways to Prevent and Deal with Lead Poisoning," from American Baby (https://www.parents.com/baby/safety/lead-poisoning/9-ways-to-prevent-and-deal-with-lead-poisoning).

State agencies: Alabama, Alaska, Arizona, Arkansas, California, Los Angeles, Colorado, Connecticut, Delaware, District of Columbia, Florida, Georgia, Hawaii, Idaho, Illinois, Chicago, Indiana, Marion County, Iowa, Kansas, Kentucky, Louisiana, Maine, Maryland, Massachusetts, Michigan, Minnesota, Mississippi, Missouri, Montana, Nebraska, Nevada, New Hampshire, New Jersey, New Mexico, New York, New York City, North Carolina, North Dakota, Ohio, Oklahoma, Oregon, Pennsylvania, Philadelphia, Rhode Island, South Carolina, South Dakota, Tennessee, Texas, Harris County, Houston, Utah, Salt Lake County, Vermont, Virginia, Washington, Seattle-King County, West Virginia, Wisconsin, Wyoming.

Get Your Free Gift.......See Page 54

Click here or visit www.leadpaintclearandsimple.com for your free gift!

Get your free copy of Kate's guide to how to identify toxins in your home and non-toxic alternatives

- Lead Paint Clear and Simple
  (http://leadpaintclearandsimple.com)

- K. Kirkwood Consulting, LLC
  (https://kkirkwood.com)

- North East Health & Housing
  (http://nehh.org)

- Lead-Edu
  (http://lead-edu.info)

- Skylar Learns About Lead Poisoning
  (http://www.skylarlearnsaboutleadpoisoning.com)

- Lead Safe Mama
  (http://www.leadsafemama.com)

9 781717 083692